DESTINY ACCORDING TO AYURVEDA

Explaining the Logic of Re-incarnation and how you can change your Destiny

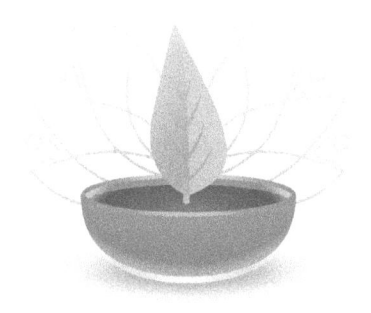

DR JAYASHREE JOSHI
M.D, D.C.H

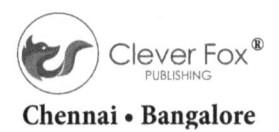

Clever Fox® PUBLISHING
Chennai • Bangalore

CLEVER FOX PUBLISHING
Chennai, India

Published by CLEVER FOX PUBLISHING 2025
Copyright © Dr Jayashree Joshi 2025

All Rights Reserved.
ISBN: 978-93-6707-900-3

This book has been published with all reasonable efforts taken to make the material error-free after the consent of the author. No part of this book shall be used, reproduced in any manner whatsoever without written permission from the author, except in the case of brief quotations embodied in critical articles and reviews.

The Author of this book is solely responsible and liable for its content including but not limited to the views, representations, descriptions, statements, information, opinions and references ["Content"]. The Content of this book shall not constitute or be construed or deemed to reflect the opinion or expression of the Publisher or Editor. Neither the Publisher nor Editor endorse or approve the Content of this book or guarantee the reliability, accuracy or completeness of the Content published herein and do not make any representations or warranties of any kind, express or implied, including but not limited to the implied warranties of merchantability, fitness for a particular purpose. The Publisher and Editor shall not be liable whatsoever for any errors, omissions, whether such errors or omissions result from negligence, accident, or any other cause or claims for loss or damages of any kind, including without limitation, indirect or consequential loss or damage arising out of use, inability to use, or about the reliability, accuracy or sufficiency of the information contained in this book.

This book is dedicated to my daughter PALASHA

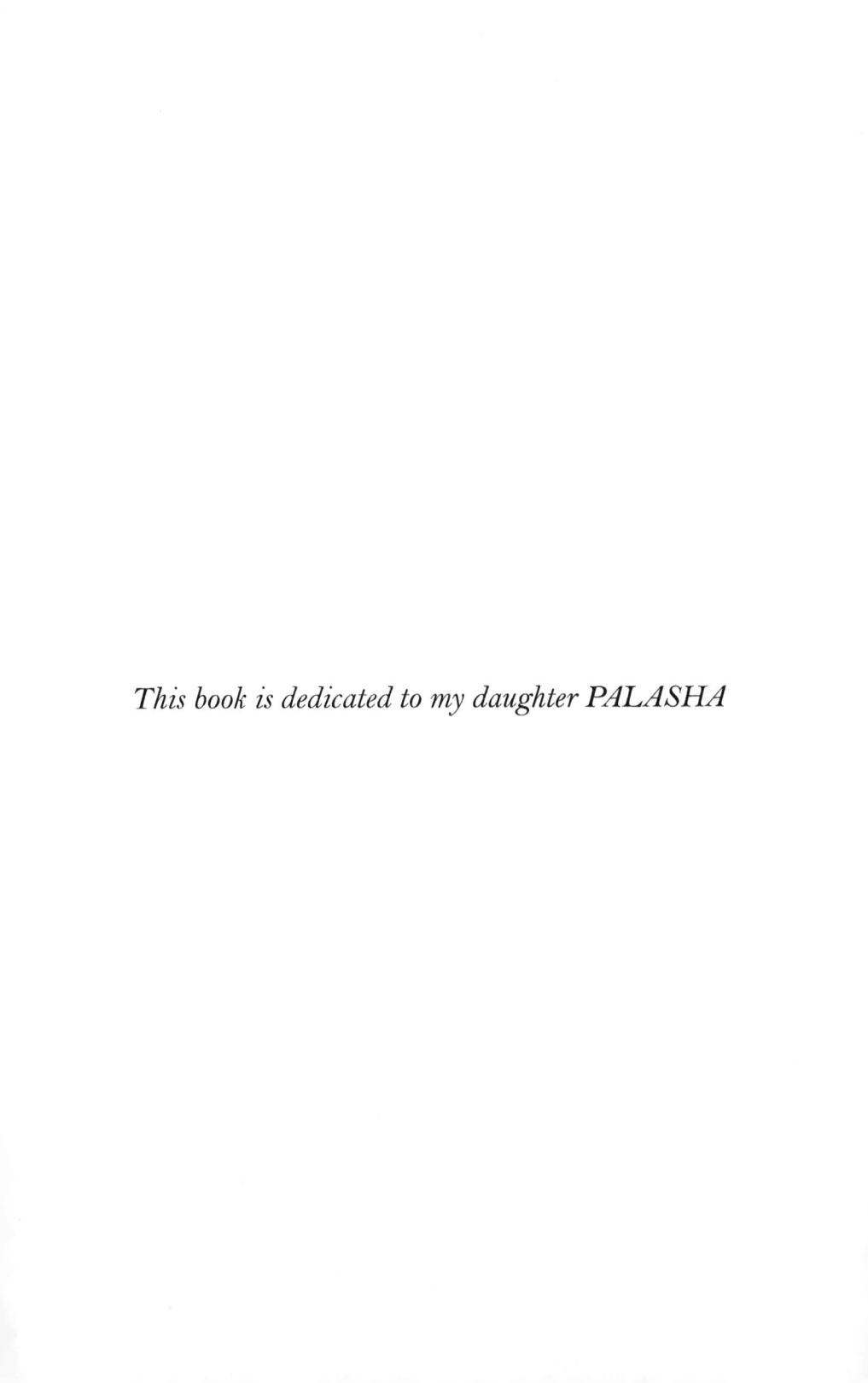

FOREWORD

*V*edic shastras, Ayurveda and Yoga are part of India's cultural heritage.

Lifestyles based on Ayurvedic principles used to be the norm in India until the arrival of modern Science which overtook and replaced many of our old habits and customs. Fortunately for me, I grew up in the languid city of Pune where traditions yet lingered and though I became a Pediatrician by formal training, I remained closely connected with Ayurveda and its Philosophy.

This book is based mostly on the *Sankhya branch* of Vedic Philosophy, from which Atharvaveda and hence, Ayurveda, are derived.

In the Epilogue of this book, I have written about how I now perceive ancient Indian philosophies when I see them through the prism of modern Medicine.

Ayurveda and modern Medicine need not be exclusive of each other. Used wisely, they can enhance the quality of a person's life, each in its own way.

The one significant difference I see between them is that Ayurveda aims to enhance the quality not only of our current life but that of our future lives as well.

Reincarnation, of course, is taken for granted in Ayurveda.

This book is addressed to followers of Vedic Philosophy.

Dr Jayashree Joshi
M.D, D.C.H
Kudal, Sindhudurg, Maharashtra
Whatsapp: 91-9834517306

CONTENTS

Foreword .... *v*

1. *WHO AM I ..... ?* 1
2. *The big Illusion called MAYA* 5
3. The Pancha koshas 6
4. Annamaya Kosha (1) 7
5. The Annamaya Kosha (2) 8
6. The Annamaya Kosha (3) 10
7. The Annamaya Kosha (4) 11
8. The Annamaya Kosha (5) 13
9. The Annamaya Kosha (6) 14
10. The Pranamaya kosha 15
11. The Manomaya kosha 17
12. Vidnynanamaya and Anandmaya Koshas 19
13. Three Doshas and Prakriti 21
14. Five types of Pitta and Five types of Kapha 23
15. Individual Prakriti 25
16. Gunas and Prakriti 27
17. Ahaar- Vihaar- Nidra 29
18. Ahaar 30
19. Vihaar 32
20. Nidra (Sleep) 33
21. Vritties 34
22. Yama and Niyama of Yoga 36
23. Epilogue 39

CHAPTER 1
WHO AM I ..... ?

*T*his is a question that occurs to most of us at some point of time.

Ayurvedic philosophy gives us *the most credible answer* to this question.

It describes the origin and structure of the Universe in detail and the function of everything it contains, going back to before even its Creation.

Ayurvedic philosophy says:

Our Universe arose due to the union of *Purush* and *Prakriti*

Purush can roughly be equated with *Consciousness* and *Prakriti* can be equated with primordial *Energy*.

Prior to their union, the Universe did not exist.

Only *the Cause* of its existence existed.

One might say here that "the Cause" / "God" / "Atma", are various nomenclatures used in accordance with different customs and beliefs.

Purush can be described as Consciousness that pervades the entire Universe.

Even objects which are not sentient are said to have some basic form of Consciousness which, of course, would be vastly different from ours.

It is important to understand that Consciousness is neither matter nor energy and the Cause (or God or Atma) is beyond even this Consciousness.

During Creation, union of *Purush* and *Prakriti* gives rise to the "big bang" (the Vedas say the Universe arises as a big bang!) and primordial Prakriti begins to manifest.

Manifestation creates *Mahat-tatwa* from which arises the *Mind Quartet*.

"Mind Quartet" means *Mind - Buddhi - Chitta - Ahankar*

From *Ahankar* of the *Mind Quartet* evolve five streams of energy called "*tanmatras* ":

Shabda tanmatra (Sound)
Sparsh tanmatra (Touch)
Rupa tanmatra (Form / Vision)
Rasa tanmatra (Taste)
Gandha tanmatra (Smell)

From evolving *Tanmatras* develop

(1) Sensory organs called *Dynanindriyas* and organs of action called *Karmendriyas*, both of which are formless.
(2) *Pancha mahabhootas,* which are made up of matter and have a physical form.

With the formation of mahabhootas, matter is formed.

The five "*Pancha mahabhootas*" are namely,

Prithvi - Aap - Tej - Vayu and *Akash*

(Earth, Water, Fire, Air and Ether).

These become the building blocks of all matter in the Universe.

During creation, matter is created from energy. The reverse occurs when the universe disintegrates.

Each mahabhoota is created by a specific tanmatra.

1. First, *Shabda tanmatra* creates *Akash* mahabhoota.
2. Next, with Akash as template, *Sparsh tanmatra* creates *Vayu* mahabhoota.
3. Then, with Vayu as template, *Rupa tanmatra* creates *Tej* mahabhoota.
4. With Tej as template, *Rasa tanmatra* creates *Aap* mahabhoota.
5. Finally, with Aap as template, *Gandha tanmatra* creates *Prithvi* mahabhoota.

Sequentially speaking,

1) Tanmatras are created from evolving primordial Prakriti
   (Tanmatras are Energies)
   and then,
2) Tanmatras create Pancha mahabhootas.
   (Pancha mahabhootas are Matter)

Energy creates Matter.

Remember Albert Einstein's famous equation, $E = mc^2$ .... ?!

"We" are created from Pancha mahabhootas and tanmatras and are infused with Consciousness.

We are always accompanied by our Atma (Soul).

CHAPTER 2

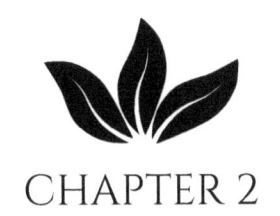

THE BIG ILLUSION CALLED MAYA

*A*yurvedic philosophy says that our *Universe* is the *macrocosm* and we are its *microcosms*.

In reality, each one of us is only a part of the whole matrix of our Universe

However, our Mind and Sensory organs, with their limited range of perception, limit us to believe and experience ourselves as separate individuals.

This is called *Maya*.

In order to understand the big illusion called *Maya*, we need to know about *Pancha koshas*.

This is what we shall see next.

CHAPTER 3

THE PANCHA KOSHAS

*A*yurveda says that our Body (or Self) has a *visible* part and an *invisible* part, although "I see you and that is You", is what we normally think.

There is a lot more to You and Me and to all of us than what we only see, for we are actually made up of five layers or *Pancha Koshas*, most of which are not even visible.

These are:

Annamaya kosha
Pranamaya kosha
Manomaya kosha
Vidnyanamaya kosha
Anandmaya kosha

Atma or Soul

Our *Atma* is said to be beyond description, definition or understanding.
It is always with us through all our lifetimes and incarnations.
It remains pure and unsullied through repetitive cycles of Life and Death.

CHAPTER 4

ANNAMAYA KOSHA (1)

Our Annamaya kosha is our *individual identity*, so to speak. It comprises our visible physical body along with our personality and other individual characteristics which belong to our invisible Inner Self.

The anatomy of the Visible body is well described in modern Medicine.

Its corresponding description in Ayurveda is a little different but is easy enough to understand and you may refer to any conventional textbook of Ayurvedic medicine to learn about it.

What we are concerned with here is the concept of the *invisible Inner Self* which is unique to Ayurvedic philosophy.

Our Inner Self is the charioteer and our visible body, the chariot.

Our Inner Self is what drives us.

Our *visible self* is the visible part of our Annamaya kosha.

It is made up of *pancha mahabhootas*.

Our *invisible Inner Self* is derived from *tanmatras* of Prakriti.

The Inner Self is our Real Self.

CHAPTER 5

THE ANNAMAYA KOSHA (2)

Pancha mahabhootas

The *Pancha mahabhootas* are five basic elements (dhatus) which co-exist in varying proportions in all (physical) matter that exists in the universe.

The dominance of respective elements in a substance determines the final quality and behavior of that particular substance.

Prithvi imparts solidity, stability, heaviness, structure and hardness.

In our body it is associated with the sense of *Smell..*

Aap imparts qualities of liquidity and fluidity, coolness, cohesion and binding.

In our body it is associated with the sense of *Taste*.

Tej gives out heat and light. It has the capacity to transform and penetrate.

In our body it is associated with *Vision*.

Vayu is in constant motion. It circulates, is ever-changing and light in weight.

In our body it is associated with the sense of *Touch*.

Akash is open space and is vast in nature. It has the capacity to hold and contain.

It transmits *Sound*.

Our Visible body is predominantly composed of *Prithvi* and *Aap* elements.

This body *keeps changing from one birth to another, through the cycle of re-incarnation.*

Our Invisible body or the *Inner Self* is composed predominantly of Energies derived from *tanmatras*, probably along with some Vayu, Akash and Tej elements.

Our Inner Self *is the cause of re-birth and it accompanies us through our cycles of reincarnation.*

Let us now understand this "Inner Self".

CHAPTER 6

THE ANNAMAYA KOSHA (3)

Our Inner Self

To put it simply, our Inner Self is the *invisible part* of our Annamaya kosha.

(There is no corresponding entity described in modern Medicine).

The *Inner Self* is composed of our:

Five Dyanindriyas

+

Five Karmendriyas

+

Mana - Buddhi - Chitta - Ahankar

(Mind - Intellect - Memory - Ego)

It is, of course, accompanied by our Soul or *Atma*

Our Inner Self is our True Self.

CHAPTER 7
THE ANNAMAYA KOSHA (4)

Dynanindriyas

Our five Dyanindriyas correspond to the five Senses described in modern Science.

Ayurveda maintains that our physical Sense Organs contain within themselves their invisible counterparts which it calls *Dyanindriyas*.

Visible Sense Organs are formed from pancha mahabhootas in the developing embryo and their *Dyanindriyas* originate from the corresponding *tanmatras* of Prakriti.

Dyanindriyas are naturally attracted to the objects of their desire, as are magnets to iron.

Hence, our eyes see things without any effort on our part, our ears automatically pick up sound waves, our nose captures smell, our tongue tastes food and our skin becomes aware of touch.

The force of attraction between Dyanindriyas and their objects is extremely strong. It cannot be easily controlled by our *Will* or Mind.

Dyanindriyas and Karmendriyas are the primary means of satisfying our Desires.

Ayurveda plays a huge role in controlling excessive Desires in our life, as we shall shortly see.

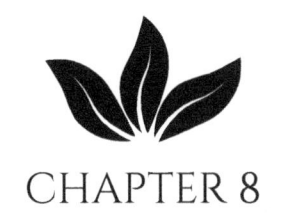

CHAPTER 8
THE ANNAMAYA KOSHA (5)

Karmendriyas

The concept of *Karmendriyas* is unique to ancient Indian Philosophies like the Vedas.

There is no parallel concept of Karmendriyas in modern Medicine.

We have *five Karmendriyas*:

Our two Upper limbs
Our two Lower limbs
Organs of Speech
Excretory organs (anus, urethra)
Genitals

Karmendriyas are *organs of action*.
Ayurveda attaches great importance to them.

CHAPTER 9

THE ANNAMAYA KOSHA (6)

The Mind Quartet

(*Mana - Buddhi - Chitta -Ahankar*)
(मन - बुद्धी - चित्त - अहंकार)

Streams of energy (called *tanmatras*) coming out from evolving Prakriti give rise to the Mind Quartet.

"Mana" means our Mind.
Conscious, Subconscious, Supraconscious and any other form that the Mind may exist in.

Buddhi is our Intellect.

Chitta refers to our awareness and memory and things connected with them.

Ahankar is our Ego.

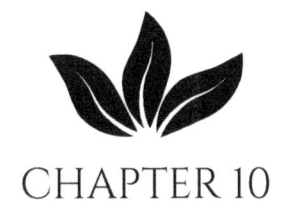

CHAPTER 10
THE PRANAMAYA KOSHA

Our Pranamaya kosha is the external sheath of the life-force which sustains us.

It is composed mainly of *Vayu* and *Akash* elements.
It extends outwards and mingles and merges with the surrounding atmosphere.

Pranamaya kosha is connected with our *five Pranas* and *Kundalini shakti* (our life-force) by means of *nadis* (nadis are yogic channels through which energy flows).
Along with five Pranas we have *five upa Pranas* as well.

Upa Pranas are sub or minor Pranas.
The five main Pranas are called *Prana, Apana, Vyana, Udana* and *Samana*.
(प्राण - अपान - व्यान - उदान - समान)

The five upa-Pranas are called *Naga, Kurma, Krikala, Devadatta and Dhananjaya*.
Prana Vayu is responsible for *inhalation* and *reception* of *sensory input*.

It is located mainly in the chest, spine and head.

Apana Vayu is responsible for elimination, excretion and downward and outward movement.

It is located mainly in the Sigmoid colon and other pelvic organs.
Vyana Vayu carries out movement, circulation and sensory perception.

It pervades the entire body.
Udana Vayu is responsible for speech, growth, and upward movement.

It is located mainly in the throat and head.
Samana Vayu governs digestion and assimilation of ingested food and nutrients.

It is located in the abdomen, mainly in the intestines.
Upa-Pranas :

Naga is responsible for belching and hiccoughs.
Kurma is responsible for blinking and the opening and closing of eyes.

Krikala is responsible for sneezing, hunger and thirst.
Devadatta is responsible for yawning.

Dhananjaya is associated with decomposition and also with the sensation of touch.
This Vayu remains in our body even after death.

CHAPTER 11
THE MANOMAYA KOSHA

*A*nd the *Mind Quartet.*
Manomaya Kosha envelopes our Pranamaya kosha
This kosha is connected with our *Mind Quartet.*
It is the realm of our thoughts, feelings and perceptions.

Mind receives sensory input from the environment through our *Dyanindriyas.*and is the primary site for processing information.
Mind is primarily said to reside in the region of our throat.

Buddhi uses intellectual power to further process this information, when required.
Buddhi is primarily said to reside near the root of the tongue.

Chitta is the site where our thoughts, experiences, emotions and perceptions reside. It is the site of memory, recall and awareness.
It is also the *storehouse of our karmic imprints.*
Chitta primarily resides in the peri-umbilical region but we can voluntarily shift Chitta to any part of our body by focusing our attention on that part.

Ahankar is where the perception of "Self" resides.
It is a perception that recognizes only our Annamaya kosha as "Self".

Ahankar resides in the heart.

Yogis say that our Manomaya kosha stretches far outwards into the earth's atmosphere and that individual manomaya koshas overlap each other.

CHAPTER 12
VIDNYNANAMAYA AND ANANDMAYA KOSHAS

Vidnyanamaya and *Anandmaya koshas* are respectively, our fourth and fifth Koshas and there is no individuality to them.

Their existence is known only to Jeevan-mukt or highly evolved Yogis. Our knowledge of these koshas comes from their teachings.

In the *Vidnyanamaya kosha*, we go beyond sensory perception into a state of greater understanding and awareness.
There we experience a *state of non-duality* and break free from the illusion of separateness created by *Maya*.

We realise the Oneness of Creation and are then able to experience the *Anandmaya kosha*, which is all-pervading *Divine Bliss* extending to the outermost reaches of the universe.
This state is called *Samadhi*.

Samadhi endows us with jeevan mukti, meaning freedom from birth and reincarnation.

"*Ekoham, Bahusyam*" is a famous quote from Brihadaranyak Upanishad.

Translated from Sanskrit, it means that the One (divine) Cause desired to experience itself in many forms. This led to creation of the universe through Purush and Prakriti.

Microcosms are formed out of the macrocosm.
We are born into the material world, in which experience of Duality (pleasure - pain / gain - loss etc) is the norm.

From one birth to another, we come under and live under the sway of our Indriyas.
Our karma multiplies, bringing Suffering in its wake.

We begin to wish that our life had been better.
Not all of us crave jeevan mukti in our current life, but we *do* hope and pray that the future will bring more joys than sorrows.

It is, indeed, possible for us to fulfill this wish.
Yoga shows us the way.
Ayurveda facilitates the journey.

On this journey we learn about *Doshas* and our *Prakriti*.

Please note:
The word "Prakriti" is used in two rather different contexts.
Until now we have used it to indicate universal primordial energy. While discussing our microcosm, the word "Prakriti" will relate to individual Constitution.

CHAPTER 13
THREE DOSHAS AND PRAKRITI

Prakriti can be equated with our *Constitution*.

Doshas are the three different outcomes of our *Ahaar, Vihaar and Nidra*.

Ahaar = food and other intake
Vihaar = activities
Nidra = Sleep or Rest
The *three Doshas* are called

Vata
Pitta
Kapha

The relative quantity / proportion of each dosha present in our body determines our Prakriti.

This proportion remains more or less constant throughout life, which means that our Prakriti also remains constant.

Doshas are composed of *pancha - mahabhootas*.

Vata dosha is formed out of *Vayu* and *Akash* pancha mahabhootas.

Vata is cold, dry and light in weight. It remains in constant motion.

In our body Vata dosha is associated with movement and the functioning of our circulatory and nervous systems.

Pitta dosha is formed out of *Tej* and *Aap* pancha mahabhootas.

Pitta is associated with heat, sharpness and intensity.

It governs digestion, assimilation and other metabolic activities and it also maintains body temperature.

Kapha dosha is formed out of *Prithvi* and *Aap* pancha mahabhootas. It is heavy, lethargic in motion and cool to touch. It gives form and stability to our body.

To stay in good health, our doshas need to remain in balance. Ayurveda teaches us how to maintain this balance through proper Ahaar- Vihaar and Nidra.

CHAPTER 14
FIVE TYPES OF PITTA AND FIVE TYPES OF KAPHA

*J*ust as there are five main types of Vayus (specific Vatas) in our body, there are five types of Pitta and five types of Kapha as well.

Five types of Pitta:

1) *Pachak pitta*
   Pachak pitta governs digestion and breaks down food into nutrients and waste.
   It is located primarily in the stomach and small intestine.
2) *Ranjak pitta*
   Ranjak pitta is involved in the formation of blood (rakta dhatu).
   It is located in the liver and spleen.
3) *Alochak pitta*
   Alochak pitta is responsible for vision and the perception of colours.
   It is located in our eyes.
4) *Sadhak pitta*
   Sadhak pitta governs our thoughts and emotions.

It is located in the heart and brain.

5) *Bhrajak pitta*

Bhrajak pitta facilitates absorption of nutrients through the skin, regulates temperature and takes care of our complexion.

It is located in the skin.

Five types of Kapha:

1) *Avalambak kapha* is located in our chest. Its function is to lubricate and nourish.
2) *Kledak kapha* is located in the stomach.
It moistens and softens ingested food and prepares the food for digestion.
3) *Tarpak kapha* is located in the head.
It nourishes the brain and Sense organs.
4) *Bodhak kapha* is located in the tongue.
It aids in the perception of taste.
5) *Shleshak kapha* is located in the joints.
It lubricates and strengthens them.

CHAPTER 15
INDIVIDUAL PRAKRITI

*E*very person possesses a unique permutation and combination of the three doshas, out of which one or two doshas tend to predominate.

The basic pattern of a person's doshas and their *relative proportion to each other* decide his Constitution.

Seven possible combinations of doshas would give the following Prakritis:

Predominantly Vata
Predominantly Pitta
Predominantly Kapha
Vata - Pitta
Kapha - Vata
Kapha - Pitta
(Since Vata - Pitta - Kapha do not exist in equal proportion, the seventh type of Prakriti remains hypothetical).

Pure Vata or pure Pitta or pure Kapha Prakritis are rarely seen.

We generally belong to a "mixed Prakriti" in which some aspects of our two main doshas tend to predominate.

Each Prakriti has different physical, mental and emotional features because the doshas have different *gunas*.

CHAPTER 16
GUNAS AND PRAKRITI

Gunas are our emotional characteristics or behavioral tendencies.

They mould our Mind and affect our Indriyas.

There are three Gunas:

Satva guna
Rajo guna
Tamo guna

Pitta dosha is associated with *Satva guna*.
It imparts *Satvik* tendencies to a person.

Vata dosha is associated with *Rajo guna*.
It imparts *Rajasic* tendencies to a person.

Kapha dosha is associated with *Tamo guna*.
It imparts *Tamasic* tendencies to a person.

Vata Prakriti is dominated by *Rajo guna*.
A Vata Prakriti person is usually thin, of slight build, has prominent veins and tendons, creaky joints, and a dry skin.

He is restless, vacillating, unpredictable and talkative, creative and quick-thinking.

He is prone to anxiety, forgetfulness, anger and aggression.

Pitta Prakriti is dominated by *Satva guna*.

A Pitta Prakriti person is of medium build, has a warm complexion with an oily skin and has a strong appetite and good digestion.
He has a sharp intellect, is sensitive, intense, passionate and competitive.
He is short-tempered, argumentative, irritable, prone to anger and is domineering.
He is spiritually oriented and inclined to be truthful.

Kapha Prakriti is dominated by *Tamo guna*.
A Kapha Prakriti person has a sturdy build, smooth skin and oily hair.
His metabolism is slow and he has a tendency to gain weight easily.
When his kapha dosha is in balance, he is a calm, composed, slow-paced, calculating and well-organized, gentle and compassionate person.
However, he is prone to being lazy, lethargic and excessively sleepy.

Excessive accumulation of any dosha results in its harmful and negative effects becoming manifest.
This leads to disease and illness.

Understanding Prakriti helps us to keep our doshas in balance through proper Ahaar- Vihaar and Nidra.

CHAPTER 17
AHAAR- VIHAAR- NIDRA

Ahaar - Vihaar and Nidra are Ayurveda's "Tripod of Health"
Ahaar = the Food we eat
Vihaar = our Activities
Nidra = our Sleep

Ahaar - Vihaar and Nidra build and sustain our body and in the process they confer certain features on us.
These features are called *Doshas*.

Doshas are a natural outcome of Ahaar - Vihaar and Nidra. Only when the quantity of any dosha exceeds its natural limit for an individual, does it cause illness.

To stay healthy in mind, body and spirit we need to control our Doshas by following the recommended Ahaar - Vihaar and Nidra for our Prakriti.

CHAPTER 18

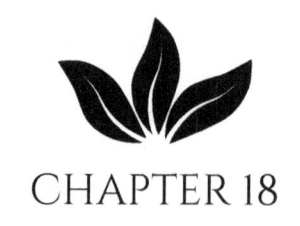

AHAAR

The food we consume contains varying combinations of six tastes, called *Rasas*.

The six Rasas or tastes are:

madhur = sweet (मधुर)
amla = sour (आम्ल)
lavan = salty (लवण)
katu = pungent (कटू)
tikta = bitter (तिक्त)
kashaya = astringent (कशाय)

Madhur rasa
Madhur rasa is associated with *Prithvi* and *Aap* mahabhootas.
It helps in nourishing and building our body,
It is heavy, oily, smooth and cold.
It increases Kapha dosha and reduces Vata and Pitta doshas.

Amla rasa
Amla rasa is associated with *Prithvi* and *Tej (Agni)* mahabhootas.
It is stimulating, warming and increases our appetite.
It is light, oily, moist and hot.
It increases Pitta and Kapha doshas and reduces Vata dosha.

Lavan rasa
Lavan rasa is associated with *Aap* and *Tej* mahabhootas.
It has heating and moisturizing properties.
It increases Kapha and Pitta doshas.

Katu rasa
Katu rasa is associated with *Tej* and *Vayu* elements.
It increases heat and dryness.
It increases Vata and Pitta doshas.

Tikta rasa
Tikta rasa is associated with *Vayu* and *Akash* elements.
It is cooling and drying in nature.
It reduces Kapha and Pitta doshas.

Kashaya rasa
Kashaya rasa is associated with *Vayu* and *Prithvi* elements.
It is drying and cooling in nature.
It reduces Kapha and Pitta doshas .

The taste of food indicates the rasas it contains. Knowledge of rasas enables us to follow a diet to suit our Prakriti.

CHAPTER 19
VIHAAR

Vihaar relates to our *activities*.

Lifestyle, daily routine, habits, behaviour and overall pattern of living .... all these and more ..... encompass Vihaar.

Our Vihaar depends on the circumstances we live in and also on our Prakriti.

Ayurveda provides guidelines of Vihaar to suit each Prakriti.

Modifying our Vihaar according to these guidelines helps us to prevent excessive accumulation of doshas.

CHAPTER 20

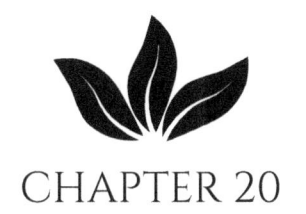

NIDRA (SLEEP)

Nidra is an essential component of life.

A person goes to sleep when his *consciousness is overcome by tamoguna.*

Our body is nourished and detoxified during sleep.
A healthy person falls asleep easily and naturally.
Growth takes place during sleep.

A person should sleep neither less nor more than is recommended for his Prakriti and should wake up feeling refreshed.

Excess kapha in a person leads to excessive sleep.
Excess Vata in a person leads to poor sleep.

Proper Ahaar and Vihaar are essential for normal Nidra.

CHAPTER 21
VRITTIES

*V*ritties *are emotions* that arise from our perceptions, says *Dynana Yoga*.

Vritties populate our Manomaya kosha and are picked up by the Mind and Senses.

They swirl in our mind and give rise to various Fears and Desires which, in turn, dictate our behavior.

raga (राग), dvesha (द्वेष), kaama (काम), krodha (क्रोध), lobha (लोभ), moha (मोह), mada (मद), matsar (मत्सर), irsha (ईर्षा), asuya (असूया), dambha (दंभ), darpa (दर्प), ahankar (अहंकार), ichcha (इच्छा), bhakti (भक्ती) and shraddha (श्रद्धा) are the major Vritties.

1. Lust, both sexual as well as for material things (राग)
2. Vengeful attitude towards someone who has hurt us in some way (द्वेष)
3. Desire to satisfy our wants (काम)
4. Anger against being contradicted (क्रोध)
5. Desire to hold on to possessions (लोभ)
6. Side-stepping discrimination (मोह)
7. Arrogance (मद)
8. Jealousy (मत्सर)
9. Wishing that ills should befall my enemies, not me (ईर्षा)

10. Benefits should be mine alone (असूया)
11. Self-glorification through deceit (दंभ)
12. Being haughty and domineering (दर्प)
13. Insisting that I am always correct (अहंकार)
14. Life-sustaining activities like hunger, thirst, excretion etc (इच्छा)
15. Following one's religious beliefs (भक्ती)
16. Believing in the tenets of one's religion (श्रद्धा)

Vritties affect us profoundly.

They are the leading cause of our *Karma*, which causes us to be born over and over again.

The first thirteen Vritties listed above lead us towards bad karma and serve to increase *tamoguna* and *rajoguna* in our Mind.

The last two Vritties listed above lead us towards good Karma and increase *satvaguna* in our Mind.

We can reduce our susceptibility to harmful Vritties by keeping our Doshas under control.

CHAPTER 22

YAMA AND NIYAMA OF YOGA

(यम and नियम) *are a set of recommendations* to be followed for overcoming harmful Vritties.

The ten Yama:

अहिंसा Ahimsa
Avoid violence in any form, whether in thought, action or speech, against any living being.

Some would say, avoid violent acts even against non-living things.

सत्य Satya
Always speak the truth, the entire truth and nothing but the truth.

अस्तेय Asteya
Do not steal or take anything from anyone without permission.

ब्रह्मचर्य Brahmacharya
Keep control over your Indriyas and especially over sexual desires.

क्षमा Kshama
Learn to forgive those who have hurt you.

धृति Dhruti
Learn to remain calm and equanimous in adverse situations.

दया Daya
Be compassionate towards everyone.

आर्जव Aarjav
Be gentle in behaviour, give up all harshness.

मिताहार Mitahar
Do not overindulge in eating.
Have satvik food.

शौच Shoucha
Keep yourself clean, physically and mentally.

The original Sanskrit shloka of the ten Yama:

"अहिंसा सत्यमस्तेयं ब्रह्मचर्यं क्षमा धृति: । दयार्जवं मिताहार: शौचं चैव यमा: दश"

The ten Niyama:

तप Tapa
Learn to ignore conflicting situations (for example, hot-cold, love-hate, gain-loss etc)

सन्तोष Santosh
Be satisfied with what you have earned and achieved.

आस्तिक्य Aastikya
Believe in a higher or divine power.

दान Daan
Donate what a recipient needs.

ईश्वर पूजन Ishwar poojan

Worship your chosen Deity / Divine Power.

सिद्धान्त श्रवण Siddhant shravan
Listen to religious and philosophical discourses.

लज्जा Lajja
Avoid shameful thoughts and acts.

मति Mati
Use your discrimination.

तप Tapa
This injunction is repeated to emphasize that achieving control over Indriyas is important.

हवन Havan
Perform all deeds with dedication and with an intent to serve.

The original *Sanskrit shloka* of the ten Niyama:

"तपः सन्तोष आस्तिक्यं दानम् ईश्वरपूजनम् सिद्धान्तवाक्यश्रवणं ह्रीमती च तपो हुतम्"

A proper regimen of Ahaar - Vihaar - Nidra increases *satvaguna* and makes Yama and Niyama look less forbidding.

Satvaguna keeps harmful Vritties at bay.

CHAPTER 23
EPILOGUE

"Ayurvedic Autonomic Nervous System"

To recapitulate, our universe is the macrocosm and we are its microcosms.

We actually exist as "a part of the whole".

But our individual Sense organs lead us to perceive ourselves as separate entities, independent of everyone else.

When we are born, energies from the macrocosm enter our body through three channels *(nadis)* in the umbilicus, carrying life-force and other energies.

These three nadis divide and subdivide into seventy-two thousand nadis which eventually enmesh our entire body.

Nadis transport *Prana* and other subtle energies to all the tissues and organs of our body and enable them to function in a cohesive and organized manner.

In addition, *nadis* also provide infrastructure upon which our Endocrine system functions.

In addition to *nadis*, there exist several fields of dense energy along the Spine, called *Chakras*.

Chakras are "wheels of spinning energy".

Seven major Chakras have been described.

From below upwards. They are:

Chakra name	Location	Function
Mooladhar	perineum	Survival
Swadhishthan	Coccyx	Procreation
Manipur	Umbilicus	Wealth, fame
Anahat	Heart	Faith / Devotion
Vishuddha	Throat	Wisdom
Agnya	Brow	non-duality
Sahasrar	Crown	Jeevan Mukti

Nadis weave in and out of these *Chakras*, carrying instructions and messages in the form of subtle energies.

Sushumna, Ida and *Pingala are nadis* which arise from *Mooladhar chakra* and *Kundalini shakti*, which is where our life-force and consciousness spring from, at the base of our Spine.

Several *Nadis* intertwine between our visible *Annamaya kosha* and invisible *Inner Self* and bind them together during life.

At the time of death *Prana vayus* exit our body, *nadis* lose their energy and the bond between our physical body and the invisible Inner Self weakens and breaks.

The visible, heavy Annamaya kosha, now lifeless, falls down.

The invisible Inner Self, which was formed from various *tanmatras*, exits the now lifeless physical body and floats freely away into the *Antariksha*, accompanied by our Atma.

Antariksha is the region of the earth's atmosphere. This is where the Inner Self stays until it is time for it to be reborn.

When it is time for it to be reborn, the Inner Self enters a pre-determined embryo and its new avatar embarks upon the journey of a new birth.

When and where and under what circumstances the Inner Self is destined to be reborn is decided by its own past Karma

Karmic record and Rebirth.

It is fascinating to conjecture how all this could be happening and *this is what I think*:

To use a modern analogy, I consider the *Chitta* as the *hardware* of the computer of a person's karmic record.

Every single action (karma) which a person performs during life is recorded on this computer.

The *Software* for recording this karma is provided by the *planets*, in the form of planetary rays and other such electromagnetic energies, which together constitute a planetary language.

Every person's karmic record accompanies and travels with his Inner Self from one birth to another, through his *Chitta*.

The person's *birth horoscope* indicates the nature of his past karma and his physical and mental characteristics in this life.

It also gives an idea of the joys, sorrows and sufferings that are now to come his way.

According to *Vedic astrology*, *Saturn* and *Rahu* are the two main karmic planets.

The designated portion of his karma which is set to unfold in the immediate future is called प्रारब्ध (pra-rab-dha). This refers to karma that has already been activated.

Activated karma cannot be altered by us alone.

We can, however, certainly attempt to modify our yet-to-be-activated karma by following the tenets of Ayurveda!

How do Prayer and Meditation work?

Of the sixteen Vritties mentioned previously, *Shraddha (Faith)* and *Bhakti (Devotion)* are said to stimulate the *Anahat chakra* (heart chakra).

Prayers, meditation and religious activities, performed sincerely, keep this *chakra* functioning in an optimal state.

I think:

Besides bestowing their conventional rewards upon a person, regular prayer / meditation lead to the release of substances similar to *Endorphins* into his blood stream.

Endorphins are hormones secreted by the Pituitary - Hypothalamic pathway of the Endocrine System.

These hormones give us an instant feeling of satisfaction and happiness.

I further think that:

It doesn't matter *Who* a person prays to, nor *What* his chosen form of meditation happens to be.

The very act of praying or meditation is, by itself, sufficient to stimulate the Anahat chakra, resulting in a release of Endorphins.

If such indeed is the case, it only validates the immortal Sanskrit *shloka* (verse):

आकाशात् पतितं तोयं यथा गच्छति सागरम्, सर्वदेवनमस्कारः केशवं प्रति गच्छति"

(Just as all water falling from the sky goes into the sea, similarly, salutations offered to all Gods go to the one and the same God)

In this shloka God is called Keshava.

I would now like to ask you, Dear Reader,

Do you agree that it makes no sense to fight over religions?

Should we not follow the tenets of Ayurveda and its philosophy to change and improve our Destiny?

                    Om Shanti! Shanti! Shanti!

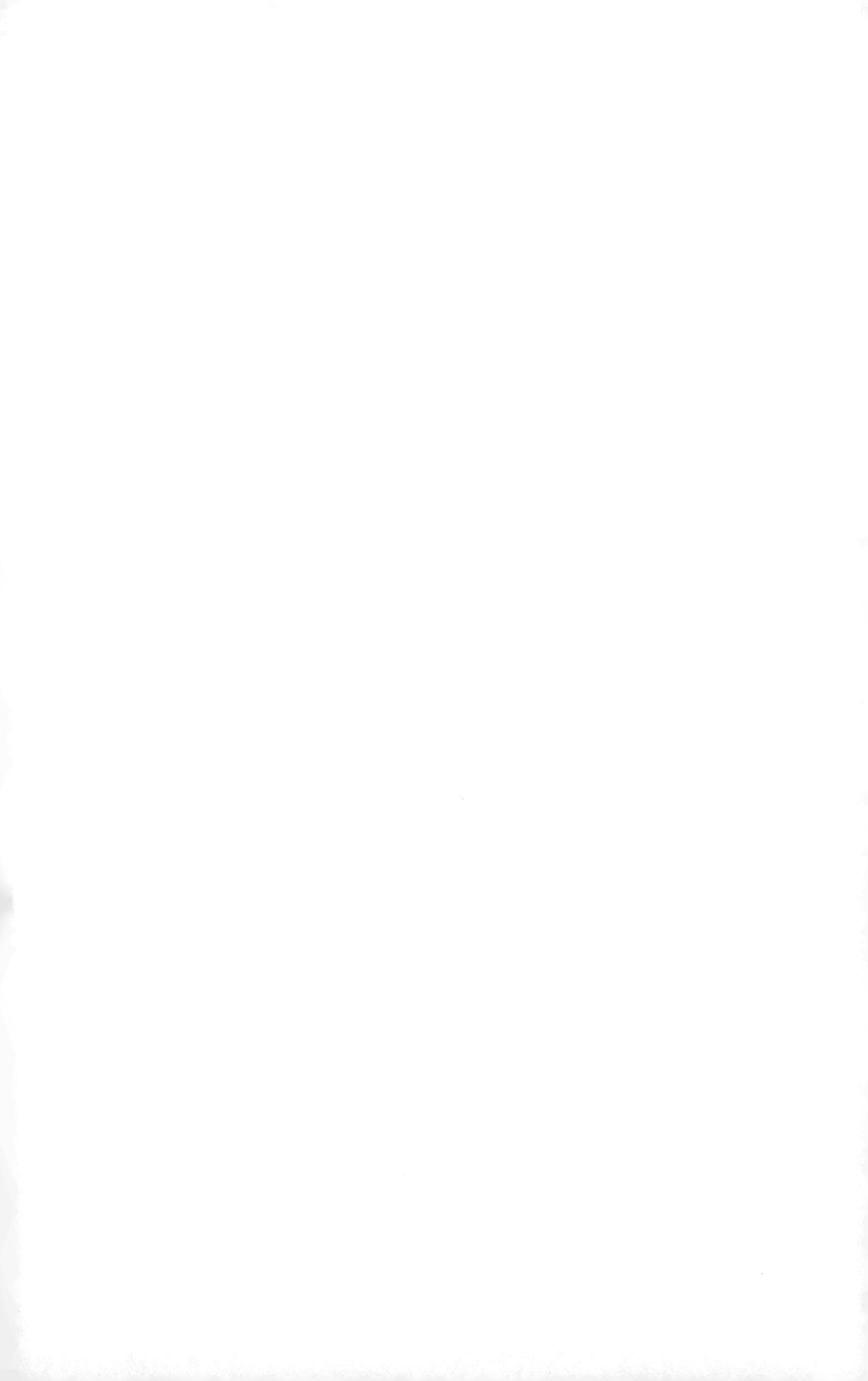